Kassandra F. Pessoa Olveira
Caroline W.S. Ferreira

Characterisation of Axillary Network Syndrome: A Cross-Sectional Study

Kassandra F. Pessoa Olveira
Caroline W.S. Ferreira

Characterisation of Axillary Network Syndrome: A Cross-Sectional Study

Post-surgical morbidities in the armpit

ScienciaScripts

Imprint

Any brand names and product names mentioned in this book are subject to trademark, brand or patent protection and are trademarks or registered trademarks of their respective holders. The use of brand names, product names, common names, trade names, product descriptions etc. even without a particular marking in this work is in no way to be construed to mean that such names may be regarded as unrestricted in respect of trademark and brand protection legislation and could thus be used by anyone.

Cover image: www.ingimage.com

This book is a translation from the original published under ISBN 978-613-9-63831-4.

Publisher:
Sciencia Scripts
is a trademark of
Dodo Books Indian Ocean Ltd. and OmniScriptum S.R.L publishing group

120 High Road, East Finchley, London, N2 9ED, United Kingdom
Str. Armeneasca 28/1, office 1, Chisinau MD-2012, Republic of Moldova, Europe
Printed at: see last page
ISBN: 978-620-7-70330-2

TABLE OF CONTENTS

SUMMARY

OBJECTIVE: To investigate axillary network syndrome (ANS), a morbidity that occurs following injury to the lymphatic vessels of the axilla as a result of surgical treatment for breast cancer. METHODS: Between December 2011 and July 2012, 97 patients surgically treated for breast cancer were enrolled, interviewed and underwent a targeted physical examination at the Cancer Hospital of Pernambuco, Brazil. All patients underwent an axillary cord test, which is characteristic of this syndrome, and shoulder joint goniometry of the ipsilateral and contralateral upper limbs. Variables on a nominal or ordinal scale were presented in the form of tables with absolute and relative frequency distributions. Variables on an interval scale were expressed as mean and standard deviation from the mean. Student's t-test was used to compare goniometric and perimetric measurements, with Lévené analysis of variance. Chi-square and Fisher's exact tests were also used to compare proportions. RESULTS: The presence of characteristic cords was diagnosed in 28.86% of the women; of the 16 women who noticed cords in the axilla, 13 (70.37%) had pain on palpation of the cords and 96.43% had a significant reduction in range of motion in passive abduction. CONCLUSIONS: SARS can only present as fibrous cords, which are not necessarily painful, but which are related to significant restrictions in the movement of the ipsilateral shoulder joint. It is therefore suggested that the clinical manifestations of the syndrome should be graded.

Keywords: Lesions of the vascular system, Axilla, Postoperative complications, Lymph node excision, Lymphatic vessels, Dissection

CHAPTER 1

INTRODUCTION: A BRIEF REVIEW OF THE SUBJECT

Neoplastic development is characterised by progressive changes in the cell's physiology, with alterations in its capacity for proliferation, differentiation, survival and interaction with the extracellular environment. It is a dynamic process that evolves in multiple stages.[37]

The term cancer is used generically to represent a group of more than 100 diseases with different localisations. An important cause of illness and death in Brazil, since 2003 malignant neoplasms have been the second leading cause of death in the population, accounting for almost 17 per cent of deaths from known causes reported in 2007 in the Mortality Information System[3] . Their global incidence continues to rise due to the ageing and increase in the world's population, as well as due to the growing adoption of behaviours that facilitate carcinogenesis in economically developing countries.[38]

Breast cancer, whose global incidence continues to rise, has a heterogeneous behaviour, with a spectrum that varies from a locoregional disease throughout its course, to a systemically disseminated disease at the time of diagnosis.[39] [41] It is probably the neoplasm most feared by women, due to its high frequency and, above all, its psychological effects, which affect the perception of sexuality and self-image.[3] It is the most common cancer among women globally. In 2008, it accounted for an estimated 23 per cent (1.38 million) of new cases and 14 per cent (458,400) of all cancer deaths worldwide[38,42] , making it the second leading cause of death. It is relatively rare before the age of 35, but from that age onwards its incidence increases rapidly and progressively.

Around half of breast cancer cases and 60 per cent of deaths occur in economically developed countries, but statistics indicate an increase in its frequency in both developed and developing countries.[38]

According to the World Health Organisation (WHO), in the 1960s and 1970s there was a 10-fold increase in age-adjusted incidence rates in Population-Based Cancer Registries on several continents. In Brazil, the estimated number of new breast cancer cases for 2012 was 52,680.[3]

The increase in breast cancer incidence observed in many countries in the 1980s and 1990s probably resulted from changes in reproductive factors (including the increased use of hormone replacement therapy), as well as due to the increased use of screening tests.[38]

Early detection of tumours by mammography and advances in medical treatment have increased patient survival[39], so that breast cancer mortality rates, once on the rise in Western countries, have been generally stable during the 1990s and, in some countries, have even declined.[43,44]

Tumour spread is an early event in breast cancer.[45] The most common sites of regional involvement in breast cancer are the axillary lymph nodes, the lymph nodes of the internal mammary chain and the lymph nodes of the supra-clavicular region. Knowledge of the likelihood of involvement of these sites and their significance is important for staging and treatment planning[8], since 70% of all breast cancer deaths occur in patients with axillary lymph node involvement at the time of diagnosis[46].

Treatment for breast cancer most often includes: surgery (sectorectomy, simple mastectomy, modified radical mastectomy), associated or not with sentinel lymph node research or axillary lymph node resection; radiotherapy, chemotherapy with anthracyclines and/or taxanes, endocrine therapy with tamoxifen or aromatase inhibitors, and anti-HER 2 therapy with trastuzumab, according to the biomarker profile of the primary tumour[47]. However, despite the therapeutic options, the main treatment is surgery, which has become increasingly refined and less invasive, especially with the advent of the sentinel lymph node technique.[48,49]

There is evidence that, following treatment for breast cancer including surgical, chemotherapy and radiotherapy modalities, biomechanical changes/deficiencies in the ipsilateral upper limb can occur twelve months to three years after treatment.[4,6]

Axillary staging is an important stage in the treatment of breast cancer, reducing the risk of axillary recurrence to less than 5% and allowing greater accuracy of prognosis and the need for adjuvant treatment.[7,50] [51] A Danish study reports that axillary lymph node involvement is present in 44% of women with breast cancer and that the percentage of lymph nodes positive for metastasis increases from 21% in tumours between 1 and 10 mm in diameter to 72% in tumours larger than 30 mm in diameter.[50]

Despite research into less invasive and less mutilating surgeries, there is still no complementary imaging test or biomarker that has been proven to be an alternative to defining the "status" of axillary lymph nodes conclusively, other than the surgical approach.[50,52]

In Brazil, as diagnoses of more advanced cases predominate, extensive surgery and axillary dissections are still widely used.[7] Such surgical management can lead to a variety of clinical morbidities that have a functional impact, but can respond to different rehabilitation interventions.[8]

The most common clinical morbidities include oedema of the chest wall and ipsilateral upper limb, impairments in the range of motion (ROM) of the shoulder joint, fibrosis of the skin, weakness in the grip strength of the hand or the strength of the shoulder girdle, shoulder stiffness, postural changes, tenderness in the chest wall, neck or in the anatomical region of the upper trapezius muscle, arm pain and numbness along the anterior aspect of the arm [78], occurring more frequently in women under the age of 65.[9,10] The incidence of these symptoms reported by women undergoing axillary dissection is 76.6%[10], with paresis being the most frequent complaint.[11]

With all the therapeutic arsenal available, women with breast cancer have a 77% chance of surviving 10 years.[53] Therefore, prevention and management of complications that can affect upper limb function should be used to improve the quality of life of patients affected by this disease, which involves not only physical aspects but also psychosocial well-being.[54]

The main psychopathological entities related to breast cancer that are present during diagnosis and treatment are: depression, fear of recurrence, sleep disorders, cognitive problems, fatigue and sexual problems. These patients are exposed to a greater risk of divorce, changes in social relationships and quality of life in general.[47]

Another disorder that is present in the pre- and post-treatment period is cancer-related fatigue. It is a prevalent symptom in advanced cancer, occurring in 75% to 95% of patients.[55,56] It is considered pathological when it persists for several months and does not diminish with rest.[55]

Factors such as a high body mass index (BMI), with a consequent increase in inflammatory substances produced by adipocytes, and in the number of leukocytes, combined with the presence of lymphoedema, can contribute to a general inflammatory state in the body, which is associated with fatigue related to " [55] cancer.

It is accepted that more conservative procedures improve patients' quality of life when compared to more radical interventions, without interfering with prognosis.[57] A study carried out in 2004 indicated that axillary dissection performed by experienced surgeons can be accompanied by minimal long-term morbidity.[58]

The initial deterioration in ipsilateral upper limb function in women who underwent axillary lymph node dissection is greater than in women who underwent sentinel lymph node biopsy.[59] Those patients who underwent complete axillary dissection are more likely to develop morbidities in the ipsilateral upper limb even without post-operative radiotherapy.[7,59-60]

On the other hand, one study reported a higher incidence of morbidities after breast-conserving surgery (sectorectomies with axillary dissection), perhaps due to the frequent association of radiotherapy in this group of patients or because preserving the thin nerve bundles is technically more difficult in smaller incisions.[30] The study by Rietman *et al.* (2003), which assessed 204 patients undergoing surgical treatment for breast cancer, showed no significant differences between morbidities in the upper limbs after axillary dissection or after sentinel lymph node biopsy.

Taking into account the nerve bundle lesions caused by surgical treatment, it can be observed that these may be a consequence of greater involvement of the axilla, which would lead to more aggressive axillary dissection and the use of radiotherapy and subsequent endocrine therapy. These procedures alone or together can cause injury to the brachial plexus.[6] The study by Leidenius *et al.* (2003) showed that sensory disorders were more common after axillary dissection, finding such alterations in 66% of patients who underwent axillary dissection and in 14% of patients who underwent sentinel lymph node examination.

The study by Johansson *et al.* (2000) found a prevalence of 89% of lesions in this plexus in women 30 years after surgery for breast cancer and in whom radiotherapy treatment had been instituted. Rõnka *et al.* (2004) observed that sensory problems in the medial aspect of the upper limb, axilla and breast were more common in patients who had undergone axillary dissection up to six months after surgery.

Hack *et al.* (1999) observed that the main symptom related to surgical treatment for breast cancer was paresthesia, which could be explained by injury to the intercostobrachial nerve during axillary lymph node dissection and the possibility of neuroma formation at the ends of the nerve. Another aspect to consider is the position of the upper limb during surgery. Breast surgery requires the ipsilateral upper limb to be in abduction, which can increase the risk of brachial plexus traction associated or not with flexion movement.[61] Post-operative brachial plexus paralysis has been reported with operative times ranging from 2 to 10 hours to periods as short as 40 minutes.[62]

Other harmful effects related to breast cancer treatment are those produced by systemic therapy. Chemotherapy agents can lead to amenorrhoea.[47,63] Also, chemotherapy together with radiotherapy to the breast or left breast plastron can cause damage to vital organs such as the heart. [6466] Other side effects such as endometrial thickening, weight gain and a decrease in bone calcium marked bone loss in patients with premature or early menopause and among postmenopausal women[47] and muscle and joint pain[9] are consequential to hormone treatment.

Another important side effect resulting from systemic treatment is peripheral neuropathies, especially as a result of the use of microtubule-stabilising agents such as paclitaxel and docetaxel, although the mechanism of their origin remains uncertain.[67] The first effects of nerve damage involve changes in electrophysiology and histochemistry. At a later stage, the findings are perineural fibrosis and injury to the vessels that irrigate these nerves.[68] Prevalence varies from low rates to 33 per cent.[67]

Chemotherapy also seems to play an important role in the development of brachial plexopathy and post-operative seroma, as well as bleeding and infection in the scar, probably because it causes perineural fibrosis.[6]

Radiotherapy can cause problems in the upper limb, such as restrictions in the mobility of the arm and shoulder. The main reasons for restricted movement are SARS and the presence of pain in the scar, surgical wound, pectoral muscle or axilla.[16] The prevalence of difficulty moving varies from less than 10% to almost 70%, depending on the assessment method (measurement or self-report), time elapsed after surgery and type of surgery, with more frequent associations with mastectomy and radiotherapy than with sectorectomies and no radiotherapy.[67]

Patients undergoing radiotherapy can present with a broad spectrum of subcutaneous fibrosis. Radiation-induced changes in fibroblast differentiation are consistent with the development of radio-induced fibrosis.[69]

Frozen shoulder syndrome (a condition of extreme difficulty in moving the shoulder joint) as a result of surgical treatment and also radiotherapy is a rare but debilitating complication that can be avoided by exercise and, when necessary, physiotherapy.[70] However, one study found incidences as high as 86% after conventional axillary lymph node dissection and 45% after sentinel lymph node biopsy.[16]

A study carried out in 2005 showed that the flexion movement of the ipsilateral shoulder joint during surgery was restricted in 34% of patients undergoing axillary dissection and 16% of patients undergoing sentinel lymph node biopsy. As for the other movements, the amplitudes were similar in these two groups.[32] Researching the same parameters, Rõnka *et al.* (2004) found a decrease in the amplitude of flexion and abduction movements of the shoulder joint after one year in 22% of women who had undergone axillary dissection compared to 10% of those who had undergone sentinel lymph node biopsy, but without statistical significance. The extent of axillary surgery did not influence external and internal rotation movements.

In addition to the aspects already discussed, it should be noted that the therapy undertaken to treat breast cancer can lead, individually or jointly, to injury of the axillary lymph nodes, with consequent interruption of the lymphatic flow in the axilla, causing lymphostasis and lowering the threshold for transmission of the nociceptive impulse, causing pain, hypersensitivity and allodynia.[20,71] Lymphostasis can lead to regional or generalised accumulation of fluids in the interstitial space, known as secondary (acquired) lymphoedema, [33,44,7273] which is the most readily recognised attribute of lymphovascular incompetence.[73]

One study suggested that an ineffective response of the lymphatic system to the stimulus provoked by physical exercise could indicate a greater risk of developing breast cancer-related lymphoedema.[74] Another investigation hypothesised that abnormalities in the (dermal) lymphatics appeared to be a consequence of lymphoedema in itself, rather than just breast cancer treatment.[75]

The study by Rõnka et al. (2005) found that patients who underwent axillary dissection reported a higher frequency of breast and upper limb oedema than patients who underwent sentinel lymph node biopsy. Another study by the same author found that one third (34.4%) of the patients surveyed (n=160) who underwent surgical treatment developed breast oedema one year after surgery.[76] These authors concluded that breast symptoms after surgery, especially lymphoedema, are significantly less common after breast-conserving surgery and sentinel lymph node biopsy than after the same surgical procedure accompanied by more extensive axillary surgery.

In particular, persistent lymphoedema over the years results in hypertrophy of the subcutaneous cellular tissue and the development of fibrosis,[77-78] characteristics which, when present, are sufficient to identify the lymphatic pathogenesis of oedema.[73]

The prevalence of lymphoedema occurring after local therapy (surgery and/or radiotherapy) varies between studies from 9.4% to 25%, one to five years after diagnosis, depending on the assessment method. ' ' ' In the majority of patients, lymphoedema occurs in the first three years after surgery. One study found that two thirds of patients developed lymphoedema in the first two years[78] ; in the following years, the incidence fell to approximately 1%.[5-47] However, the prevalence of lymphoedema can be overestimated when self-reports obtained through questionnaires are taken into account, since sensory disorders such as paresis or paresthesia can be perceived by patients as lymphoedema.[16]

Factors that can influence the development of secondary lymphoedema in the ipsilateral upper limb are the number of lymph nodes removed, radiotherapy in the armpit, ' ' ' surgical wound infection, post-surgical drainage time, immobility of the ipsilateral limb, obesity and skeletonisation of the axillary vein.[70]

In one study, obesity and infection/injury were the predictive factors most statistically associated with lymphoedema.[58] The importance of BMI as a predictor of oedema in the limb contralateral and ipsilateral to the surgery was corroborated by the finding that women with a higher body mass index had higher rates of oedema in the affected upper limb.[10] Another study found that very thin skin flaps with removal of subcutaneous tissue lymphatics and extensive incisions can contribute to the genesis of lymphoedema.[83]

As for the clinical diagnosis of lymphoedema, the most commonly used method is to compare the circumference of the upper limbs measured by a tape measure. Measuring more than one location is important as the shape of the limbs can differ between individuals before and after lymphoedema, as well as within the same individual. There is no standard measurement, but a 2cm difference between the arms is the most widely accepted parameter.

Other morbidities that occur after breast cancer surgery are seromas, haematomas and infections. Obesity can be a facilitating agent for these problems. A review article showed moderate evidence of how individuals with a higher body weight undergoing radical mastectomy are more susceptible to seroma formation and a drainage time of more than three days, when compared to those undergoing simple mastectomy.[84]

It has been proposed that low levels of fibrinogen and the activity of the fibrinolytic network in lymphatic fluids contribute to seroma formation.[23] In addition, it is known that the sectioning of lymphatic vessels during surgery leads to its late formation, but its aetiology has not yet been fully elucidated.[85] Its incidence can be as high as 50 per cent when the time spent using an axillary drain is shortened.[86] The closed spaces of breast surgery cavities, surgical scars and the cavity between the anterior chest wall and the skin of the mastectomy site are the main sites of seroma accumulation.[23]

With regard to the presence of haematoma as a complication following breast surgery, it can be seen that its incidence has been drastically reduced by the routine use of electrocautery, but this complication continues to occur in 2% to 10% of cases.[87]

Recurrent episodes of breast cellulitis, occurring several months to years after quadrantectomy and/or radiotherapy, have an incidence of around 5% of patients, but this uncommon and late complication causes significant concern because of the need to exclude inflammatory breast carcinoma. The cause of the late onset of breast oedema and cellulitis is incompletely understood, but the presence of lymphatic obstruction, which affects intramammary drainage, is accepted. Risk factors for these conditions include a history of post-operative complications such as haematoma and seroma, upper limb lymphoedema and breast surgeries with removal of a larger volume of glandular tissue.[23]

With regard to the pain symptoms that occur during and after treatment for breast cancer, it was observed that 92% of the patients with onset of pain complaints in the ipsilateral upper limb within twelve months had received radiotherapy.[5] According to Gãrtner et al. (2009) 47% of women who have received treatment for breast cancer report pain in the region of the surgery 1 to 3 years after the end of treatment.

The incidence of chronic pain seems to be higher in young women, with a more advanced primary clinical stage and who had complained of more severe pain in the immediate post-operative period.[29,30] Chronic upper limb pain was also associated with tumour invasion of the axillary lymph nodes and endocrine treatment. Risk factors for this symptom include younger age, larger diameter tumours, undergoing radiotherapy and chemotherapy, depression and impaired defence mechanisms.[23]

Complaints of pain tend to diminish over time, but persist in around 20 per cent of patients three years after surgery.[47] One study showed that 47 per cent of women treated for breast cancer reported pain, 58 per cent reported sensory disturbances in the area of the surgery one to three years after treatment, and half of the women reported moderate to severe pain.[9]

With the evolution from more radical surgeries to conservative surgeries, which have become the standard for the treatment of early-stage breast cancer[57] , it has been observed that chronic pain also occurs after sectorectomy or quadrantectomy,[7] with a reported incidence of 10.8 per cent of this symptom after conservative surgeries.[10]

Steegers *et al.* (2008) found a 23 per cent prevalence of chronic pain without classic axillary lymph node dissection and 51 per cent with lymph node dissection. Some studies have observed that complaints of upper limb pain were more common after axillary dissection than after sentinel lymph node biopsy.[32,71] Leidenius *et al.* (2005) reported that 40% of patients who underwent sentinel lymph node biopsy and 13% of patients who underwent axillary dissection were completely free of symptoms in the ipsilateral upper limb three years after surgery.

The study by Hack *et al. in* 1999 found that complaints of pain were significantly more associated with the number of lymph nodes dissected. An association between the complaint of pain and the location of the tumour in the upper quadrant was not found in the study by Gãrtner *et al.* (2009).

Pain after surgery for breast cancer can result from damage, usually transient and self-limiting, to the muscles and ligaments or it can affect the nerve tissue, which would prolong the symptom.[88] A minority of breast cancer patients experience chronic incisional pain, which can be debilitating, refractory to analgesics and last for months or years after surgery.[23]

The most common cause of pain after mastectomy is trauma to the intercostobrachial nerve. [29,89] This nerve, which is often injured during axillary dissection, also leads to the appearance of paresthesia. The skin supplied by the severed nerve appears to have altered thermoregulation and is therefore susceptible to injuries such as burns.[90] According to research by Gãrtner *et al.* (2009), chronic pain following surgery and adjuvant therapy for breast cancer can be characterised as a "neuropathic pain state" and results from damage to the intercostobrachial nerve. The fact that the incidence and intensity of pain in the ipsilateral upper limb maintained a significant correlation with the incidence of paresthesia, oedema, "phantom" sensations and muscle weakness confirms the nerve injury.[30]

Another explanation for the pain in the upper limb could be reflex sympathetic dystrophy, also known as *complex regional pain syndrome* (CRPS), an alteration of a region of the body, usually the extremities, characterised by pain, oedema, limited range of movement, vasomotor instability, skin changes and uneven bone demineralisation.[89]

Radiation-induced plexopathy, i.e. radioactive neuritis, is also a well-known cause of chronic pain.[91] Axillary dissection and radiotherapy were significantly more associated with the presence of pain regardless of the surgical procedure (mastectomy or conservative surgery) or the use of chemotherapy.

Chemotherapy and radiotherapy do not seem to be related to the presence of chronic scar pain,[6] . However, Gãrtner *et al.* (2009) found a strong association between chemotherapy and reports of pain as well as sensory disturbances in the upper limb ipsilateral to the surgery and in the operated breast area, when they used univariate analysis. This effect disappeared when multivariate analysis was used.

Post-operative bleeding/hematomas seem to have a greater association with the presence of scar pain, probably due to the fibrosis resulting from these pathological processes.[30]

One of the main causes of post-operative pain and one that is probably related to the surgical treatment of breast cancer with an axillary approach is axillary network syndrome (ANS), which is characterised by the development of cord-like structures in the medial and upper portion of the arm and over the anterior portion of the elbow, a finding that is a fundamental condition for diagnosing the syndrome,[9] which can extend proximally along the lateral chest wall.[12]

The incidence of axillary network syndrome, also known as cord[12] or cord lymphoedema[8] is still not well defined.[12] It has a variable incidence of 6%,[17] 28.1%,[14] 38.2%,[13] 42.3%,[16] up to 48.3%,[15] according to the few reports in the literature, given its vague definition.[18]

Its incidence, in terms of the type of surgical approach in the axilla, varies between 36% in women who underwent axillary dissection and 11.7% when sentinel lymph node research was carried out.[14] However, SARS, observed after sentinel lymph node biopsy (after sentinel lymph node examination, there is a reported incidence of 10%[16] has been less severe and is limited to the axilla and medial aspect of the arm, without extending to the wrist.[17]

Moskovitz *et al.* (2001) observed that SARS did not seem to be associated with the presence and number of positive lymph nodes on axillary dissection. However, another study found that women with positive lymph nodes on histopathological examination had a 62% higher risk of developing SARS than women without axillary lymph node metastases.[14]

SARS is an important self-limiting cause of axillary surgery morbidity, occurring not only in the immediate postoperative period.[15] The onset of symptoms occurs one to two weeks after surgery, with spontaneous resolution in two to three months.[12][15] However, this aspect is also the subject of controversy, as some authors have reported the appearance or return of SARS months or even years after surgery.[15][16]

Studies have found a lower average age for patients with SARS than patients without SARS.[14][15] This could be related to BMI, since older people tend to gain more weight due to a natural decrease in metabolism.[15]

The SRA is more prominent in slim patients, perhaps due to the thickness of the subcutaneous cellular tissue, since in patients with thick subcutaneous cellular tissue the detection of the network can be difficult, as well as making it difficult to adhere the skin to the underlying tissues provided by the cords.[12]

This syndrome is characterised by the presence of an axillary network that is mostly visible on post-operative physical examination (Figure 1.1), when patients try to abduct their arms, ' ' by pain originating in the axilla ' and/or the olecranon, radiating to the lower portion of the ipsilateral arm, causing limited shoulder movement and elbow extension ' leading to changes in movement patterns.

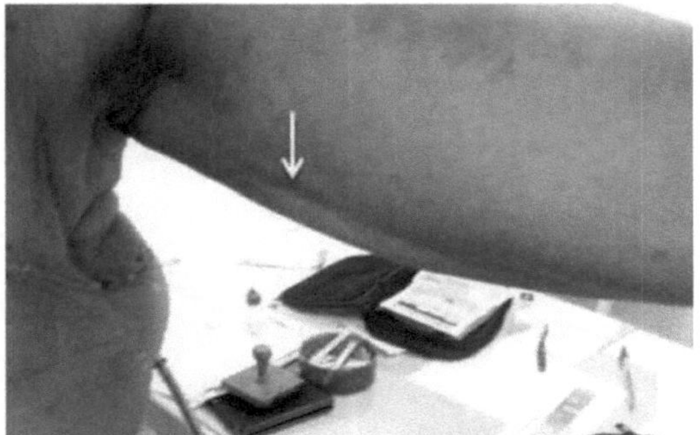

Axillary hammock syndrome (personal collection)

The cords usually break spontaneously or during a treatment session when the therapist applies manual traction to them. These structures do not bleed after they are broken.[8] They can be observed by the skin retracting or sometimes moving towards the ipsilateral upper limb; a protrusion or retraction of the skin is seen near the venous vessels depending on the thickness of the skin.[24]

It is recognised that these fibrous bands may be sclerosed lymphatic vessels[8,21] and the term "occlusive thrombotic lymphangiofibrosis" was suggested by Marsch *et al.* (1986). SARS can be suggested as a variant of Mondor's Syndrome, i.e. a benign thrombophlebitis of the superficial veins of the breast[22], since the typical symptoms of this syndrome are the presence of one or more palpable and painful cords in the subcutaneous tissue.[23] The incidence of breast cancer in association with Mondor syndrome is 11.7 per cent. [24]

Cord biopsies of a small number of patients show dilated lymphatics, venous thrombosis and fibrosis in the lymphatics. Thus, pathological and anatomical evidence contributes to supporting the angiolymphatic origin of SARS. The observation of fibrin clots in superficial veins and in lymphatic vessels of axillary networks that were biopsied suggests that lymphovenous trauma, stasis and hypercoagulability are implicated in the genesis of the syndrome. Thus, the removal of axillary lymph nodes would lead to SARS by various mechanisms.[17]

The lymphatic vessels would suffer an injury that would obstruct the flow of lymph,[12][17] which would lead to thrombosis, resulting in inflammation, fibrosis and shortening of the tissues. In addition, the tissue injury caused during surgery would release the tissue factor, which could cause hypercoagulability in adjacent tissues.[17] However, although lymphatic thrombosis seems to be more common, venous thrombosis, especially deep vein thrombosis (DVT) of the upper limb, is an uncommon entity. The main aetiologies include primary thrombosis related to stress or exertion, surgical or accidental trauma, venous channelling, chemical or infectious thrombophlebitis, thoracic outlet syndrome, congestive heart failure, uremia, vasculitis, thrombocytosis, polycythaemia[94] and malignant neoplasms.[23][94]

In view of the above, axillary lymph node dissection, sentinel lymph node dissection, trauma, or obstruction due to the cancer itself,[12,16,92] as well as lymphovenous trauma that occurs when the tissue is retracted and when the patient is positioned during axillary lymph node dissection[17] may be implicated in the genesis of SARS.

Among the contributing factors to vascular diseases, the contribution of smoking and diseases such as diabetes mellitus (DM) and systemic arterial hypertension in the genesis of SARS does not yet seem to be known, however, it is described in the literature that all three conditions are present in the etiology of micro and macrovascular complications.[95]

Smoking causes well-established vascular damage as it accelerates and aggravates atherosclerosis and increases the risk of coronary artery disease. Nicotine stimulates the release of catecholamines, stimulates damage to the arterial endothelium and promotes atherogenesis.[96]

Smokers have alterations both in the biological vascular balance, which favours thrombogenesis through effects on platelets and coagulation factors, and in the vascular tone balance, which favours vasoconstriction. Smoking also potentiates thrombosis in endothelial dysfunction by increasing the plasma concentration of fibrinogen and altering platelet activity.[96] Nicotine and other components of cigarettes have well-known side effects on the small vessels of the skin, resulting in an approximate four-fold increase in the risk of skin infection after breast surgery.[23]

Type 2 diabetic patients, on the other hand, are four times more likely to have peripheral vascular disease and cerebral vascular disease. Some factors that, together with diabetes mellitus, lead to vascular complications are mainly hypertension, dyslipidaemia, smoking, as well as endothelial dysfunction, pro-thrombotic state and inflammation.[95]

Another aspect also observed was the association between SARS and other morbidities following axillary surgery. In one study, women with an increase in upper limb volume (> 200 ml) in the first six months after axillary dissection had a 1.54 times greater risk of SARS compared to those with normal volume.[13] Another study, which assessed the effectiveness of physiotherapy in preventing the presence of lymphoedema after axillary dissection in breast cancer surgeries, found that among 18 patients who developed secondary lymphoedema, 12 presented with ARS in the second and third week after surgery,[15] while another study (Moskovitz *et al.*, 2001) found a concomitant 11%. In contrast, Bergmann *et al.* (2012) found no association between the occurrence of lymphoedema and SARS, but when it came to the sensation of oedema (subjective oedema) there was an almost twofold increase in the risk of developing SARS.

Regarding the occurrence of post-surgical healing complications, it was observed that the presence of haematomas was statistically associated with SARS, doubling its risk. Surgical injury to the intercostobrachial nerve (clinically translated as the presence of paresis) increased the risk of developing SARS threefold.[14]

Despite what has been said about the aetiological and associated factors, long-term sequelae have not been identified in SARS patients (Moskovitz *et al.*, 2001), and spontaneous regression has been observed 12 weeks after onset (Reedijk *et al.*, 2006).

The exact origin, presentation and clinical evolution, as well as the treatment of SARS still need to be better elucidated[25,26] and despite the use of non-hormonal anti-inflammatory drugs or opioids for pain management[97] there is a lack of formal guidelines on which to base therapeutic interventions.[25]

CHAPTER 2

MATERIALS AND METHODS

Data collection was carried out at the Pernambuco Cancer Hospital (HCP) as it is a place with a high demand for oncological surgery. The study population consisted of patients seen at the hospital's Mastology Department outpatient clinic between December 2011 and July 2012. The study design was cross-sectional, observational, analytical with comparison of groups, relating to anamnesis of symptoms reported in the ipsilateral upper limb after the surgical event and collection of axillary network syndrome data to meet the objective of this study.

To determine the sample sizei (N), the incidence of axillary mesh syndrome was assumed to be 28.1%, as reported by Bergmann *et alS[14]* \ because it was the only recent Brazilian study to determine this parameter, and 6%, as reported by 17 *et [alSIT]* because it was the lowest incidence found and the first reported. This percentage was applied to the Whitley and Bali formula[27] . The N then ranged from approximately 94 patients (for a significance level of 0.05 and power of proof equal to 90 per cent) to 162 patients (for a significance level of 0.01 and power of proof equal to 95 per cent). Data was collected from 131 patients, which corresponded to a power of proof equal to 99.3% (for a significance level of 0.05). After applying the exclusion criteria, the sample consisted of 97 patients.

The inclusion criteria were: female gender, age equal to or greater than 18 years, attendance at the Mastology outpatient clinic at the Pernambuco Cancer Hospital between December 2011 and July 2012, diagnosis of unilateral breast cancer. The exclusion criteria were: diagnosis of recurrent unilateral breast cancer; no record of breast cancer diagnosis in the medical records; more than two sessions of physiotherapy treatment in the ipsilateral upper limb after breast cancer surgery.

Sample constitution flowchart (STROBE model):

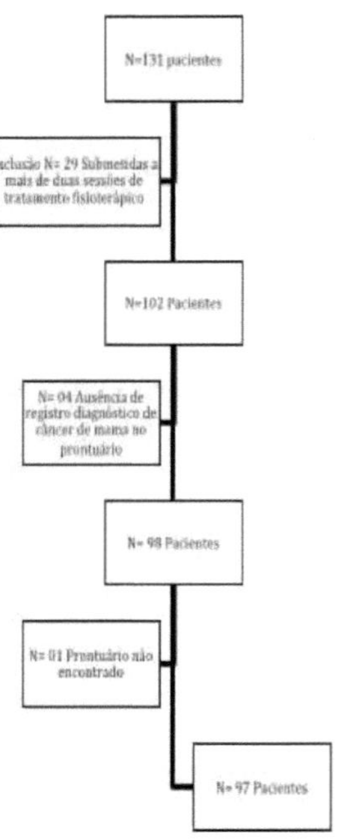

The predictor variables were: age, breast laterality; self-report of pain in the upper limb ipsilateral to the committed breast (symptom); self-report of pain in the surgical scar (symptom); pain on palpation of the cords (sign) - Pain complaints were classified as mild, moderate or severe, assessed by the visual analogue scale - VAS - self-report of weakness in grip/hand grip (symptom); self-reported paresis (symptom); self-reported paresthesia (symptom); altered active and passive range of motion (ROM) of the shoulder joint using goniometry, which consisted of measuring the maximum angle of the shoulder joint ipsilateral and contralateral to the affected breast, expressed in degrees. Active movements were measured - when the patient performed them herself - and passive movements - when the examiner helped her perform them. The movements assessed were flexion, extension, abduction, adduction, external and internal rotation of the ipsilateral and contralateral shoulder joint.

For this study, altered range of motion was considered to be a reduction of 10° or more in the goniometry of the limb ipsilateral to the surgery, compared to the contralateral limb. The outcome variable was the presence of cords in the axilla (sign) - Presence of SARS. All patients were assessed using the same goniometer (CARCI®-360°).

After inviting each patient to take part in the research, they were given a Free and Informed Consent Form. This was followed by the application of a questionnaire to record complaints related to breast cancer treatment. Active and passive goniometry was carried out on both upper limbs and axillary cord research was carried out on the upper limb ipsilateral to the surgery, the data from which was recorded on the same questionnaire.

The data was organised in an *Excel®* spreadsheet and analysed using the *Statisticcil Pctckcige for Social Sciences* (SPSS®) software, version 20.0.

Variables on nominal or ordinal scales were presented in the form of tables with absolute and relative frequency distributions. Quantitative variables on an interval scale were expressed as mean and standard deviation from the mean.

To compare the goniometric measurements of the limbs ipsilateral to the breast lesion with those of the contralateral limbs, Student's t-test was used for differences in means of paired data, with Lévené analysis of variance, since each patient was her control. Chi-square and Fisher's exact tests were also used to compare proportions. A significance level of 0.05 was adopted for all inferential tests.

The tables were constructed in accordance with the tabular presentation standards of the Brazilian Institute of Geography and Statistics[28] .

The research was approved by the Ethics Committee for Research Involving Human Beings of the Pernambuco Cancer Hospital, under registration CAAE 03260172447- 11. All the recommendations of Resolution 196/96 of the National Health Council were complied with, including the rights of the patients and the duties of the researcher.

CHAPTER 3

RESULTS

Characteristic SARS cords were identified in 28 patients (28.86%). Table 1 shows the associations between symptoms related to breast cancer surgery and the diagnosis of SARS. It was found that pain in the surgical scar, pain in the upper limb ipsilateral to the surgery, as well as reports of the perception of cords were significantly associated with the presence of ARS. There was a predominance of reports of paresis in the upper limb ipsilateral to the surgery and limited shoulder movement, regardless of the presence of ARS. Pain on palpation of the cords was present in 70.37% of the women who reported the perception of cords.

In order to detail the occurrence of symptoms related to breast cancer surgery, the means and standard errors of the mean age of the patients were determined according to the occurrence of ARS, which revealed a significant association between all the complaints investigated and the presence of ARS, with the exception of the report of the perception of painful cords. There was also a younger mean age for almost all the complaints investigated in women with ARS (Table 2).

As for the characteristic cords of SARS, there was a predominance of pain on palpation on physical examination, with mild to moderate intensity, as shown in Graph 1.

Table 3 shows the frequency distribution of reduced active and passive shoulder movement in patients with axillary network syndrome, according to the presence of pain on palpation of the cords. There was a predominance of reduced movement unrelated to the presence of pain on palpation for all active and passive movements, with the exception of active external shoulder rotation.

Table 4 shows that most of the women, regardless of the presence or absence of SARS, had reduced active and passive shoulder movement, with no difference between the groups. The most frequent impairments occurred in active and passive flexion, active and passive abduction and passive internal rotation of the shoulder. It should be noted that the only reduction in movement with a significant difference between the groups was passive shoulder abduction, which was more frequent among women with SARS (96.46%).

CHAPTER 4

DISCUSSION

With regard to the criteria for diagnosing the syndrome, research suggests palpation or visualisation of the cords, as well as an association with the presence of pain on palpation or reduced range of movement of the limb ipsilateral to the affected breast, but these criteria are not usually described in detail, making it impossible to compare the frequencies more accurately[13,17].

It is interesting that complaints of pain in the axillary region were not restricted to patients with RAS; they were common in them, but also in patients without RAS, and these complaints may be more related to the postoperative state *per se* than to the presence of the syndrome. The wide variation in pain reported by the women included in this study may be due to different concepts of pain, i.e. different individual interpretations, and different types of surgical and adjuvant treatment used[9].

The proximity between data collection and surgical treatment also seemed to explain why the higher frequency of reports of limited shoulder movement, paresis in the ipsilateral upper limb and perception of painful cords, although frequent in women diagnosed with the syndrome, were also common in those without the syndrome. This observation was not mentioned in the literature consulted, which is relevant given the scarcity of studies on SARS.

The lack of an association between these symptoms and ARS may have been due to the choice to collect data close to the surgical treatment, i.e. the inclusion of women who had not had more than two physiotherapy appointments. Considering that the local service in this study routinely institutes physiotherapy treatment immediately, we tried to minimise the influence that physiotherapy could have on the evolution of morbidities in the post-operative period, acting as a confounding factor. However, this strategy could explain the greater association of symptoms with the post-operative recovery period. Perhaps a longer follow-up of these patients could elucidate these associations.

As for the physical examination, the relationship between the presence of characteristic SARS cords and pain on palpation was in line with that proposed by several authors[15 17] since this symptom is part of the triad attributed to axillary network syndrome: the presence of cords originating in the axilla, pain on palpation and a deficit in the range of movement of the shoulder joint. However, it should be noted that pain was not present in all cases, which leads us to reflect on the existence of incomplete ARS.

The significant difference in age between the group of women with SARS and without SARS in terms of complaints of axillary pain, limited shoulder movement, paresthesia, paresis and decreased strength in the ipsilateral upper limb corroborated the findings of several studies of a higher prevalence of complaints and post-surgical morbidities diagnosed in the younger population 29-30) gm $_{se}$ tratanj$_0$ j$_{as}$ complaints, This could be explained, in part, by the observation that symptoms such as depression, anxiety, hostility and anger are more common in the younger population and, as such, exacerbate the impact that the surgical treatment and its aftermath would have on their daily lives[31] .

The association between pain on palpation of the cords and reduced range of movement was frequent and was in line with reports in the literature[15, 17] . This association may have several possible explanations, among which are the muscle injury itself, the fear of movement after surgery, the physiology of the healing process consisting of mechanical impediment to movement and the very presence of SARS cords. Further cohort studies with prolonged follow-up are needed to prove these hypotheses.

The main limitation of this study was its cross-sectional nature, i.e. the fact that the patients were not followed up over time, so conclusions could not be drawn about the causality of factors associated with axillary network syndrome. Also, its retrospective stage is in itself a limitation, since obtaining information written by third parties and self-reporting symptoms experienced in the past by the patients themselves can lead to interpretation and memory biases.

This study did not assess the patients prior to surgery, as in some studies[9,32, 34]0 which may have hindered the detection of range of motion deficits and differences in upper limb circumference prior to surgery.

An attempt was made to minimise this inconvenience by comparing the upper limb ipsilateral to the surgery with its contralateral limb. The contralateral limbs do not seem to show any apparent changes from a clinical point of view, which validates the methodological approach adopted - -,93235 \ however, as demonstrated in the review by Fukushima *et alS*[36] \ the contralateral upper limbs may also undergo adaptive haemodynamic changes after the traumatic event (axillary dissection).

In view of the above, it can be concluded that SARS may only present as fibrous cords, which are not necessarily painful, but which are related to a significant restriction in the movement of the ipsilateral shoulder joint. It is therefore suggested that SARS could be defined by a gradation of clinical manifestations that could vary in type and intensity, with the common point being the presence of fibrous cords.

CHAPTER 5

ACKNOWLEDGEMENTS

We would like to thank Drª Lais Guimarães Vieira for her valuable contribution to the statistical analysis and interpretation of the data.

REFERENCES

1. Siegel R, Naishadham D, Jemal A. Cancer statistics. 2012 American Cancer Society. CA: Cancer J Clin. 2012;62:10-29.

2. Canadian Cancer Society's Steering Committee On Cancer Statistics 2012. Canadian cancer statistics 2012. Canadian Cancer Society. 2012;71 -74.

3. Brazil. 2012 Estimate: Cancer Incidence in Brazil. Inca. General Coordination of Strategic Actions. Coordination of Prevention and Surveillance. 2011:118.

4. Bentzen SM, Dische S. Morbidity related to axillary irradiation in the treatment of breast cancer. Acta Oncol 2000;3:337-47.

5. Springer BA, Levy E, Garvey C, et al; Preoperative assessment enables early diagnosis and recovery of shoulder function in patients with breast cancer. Breast Cancer Res Treat *Volume 120*. 2010;l: 135-147.

6. Tasmuth T, Smitten K, Kalso E. Pain and other symptoms during the first year after

radical and conservative surgery for breast cancer. Br J Cancer 1996;74:2024-2031.

7. Ferreira BPS, Pimentel MD, Santos LC *et al.* Morbidity between sentinel lymph node post-biopsy and axillary dissection in breast cancer. Rev Assoe Med Bras São Paulo 2008;6: 517-21.

8. Hellman S, Harris J R. Natural History of Breast Cancer. In: Diseases of the Breast. 2nd edition. São Paulo: Medsi, 2002: 489-508

9. Gârtner R, Jensen M B, Nielsen J, et al; Prevalence of and factors associated with persistent pain following breast cancer surgery. JAMA. 2009;302:1985-92.

10. Yap KP, McCready DR, Narod S, et al. Factors influencing arm and axillary symptoms after treatment for node negative breast carcinoma. Cancer. 2003;96:1369-1375.

11. Hack TF, Cohen L, Katz J, et al. Physical And Psychological Morbidity After Axillary LymphNode Dissection For Breast Cancer. J Clin Oncol. 1999;1:143-149.

12. Koehler L A. Axillary Web Syndrome. Lymphedema Management: The Comprehensive Guide for Patients and Practitioners. 2. ed. New York, NY: Thieme Medical Scientific Publishers. 2009;70-72.

13. Bergmann A, Mattos IE, Pedrosa E, et al; Axillary web syndrome after lymph node

dissection: results of 1004 breast cancer patients. Lymphology. 2007;40 (suppl): 198-203.

14. Bergmann A, Mendes VV, Dias RA, et al; Incidence and risk factors for axillary web syndrome after breast cancer surgery. Breast Cancer Res Treat 2012; 131 (3):987-992.

15. Lacomba MT, del Moral OM, Zazo JLC, et al; Axillary web syndrome after axillary dissection in breast cancer: a prospective study. Breast Cancer Res Treat 2009;117(3):625-630.

16. Leidenius M, Leppãnen E, Krogerus L, et al; Motion restriction and axillary web syndrome after sentinel node biopsy and axillary clearance in breast cancer. Am J Surg. 2003;185:127-130.

17. Moskovitz AH, Anderson BO, Yeung RS, et al;. Axillary web syndrome after axillary dissection. Am J Surg. 2001;181:434-439.

18. Tilley A, Maclean RT, Kwan W. Lymphatic cording or axillary web syndrome after breast cancer surgery. Can J Surg. 2009;4:E105- EI06.

19. Marcus RT, Pawade J, Vella J. Painful lymphatic occlusion following axillary lymph node surgery. 1990. Br J Surg;77:683.

20. Cheville AL, Tchou J. Barriers to rehabilitation following surgery for primary breast cancer. J Surg Oncol. 2007;5:409-418.

21. Marsch WCh, Haas N, Sttittgen G. Mondor's phlebitis'- A lymphovascular process. Dermatologica. 1986;3:133-138.

22. Dixon, J.M. Erythematous Disorders Of The Breast. Available at: <Http://Www.Uptodate.Com/Contents/Erythematous-Disorders-Of-The-Breast?Source=Search_Result&Search=Mondor+Breast+Disease&Selectedtitle=1%7

el 50> Accessed on 22/08/2012.

23. Vitug AF, Newman LA. Complications in breast surgery. Surg Clin North Am. 2007;87:431-51.

24. Catania S, Zurrida S, Veronesi P, et al. Mondor's disease and breast cancer. Cancer. 1992;69:2267-7220.

25. Fourie WJ, Robb KA. Physiotherapy Management of Axillary Web Syndrome Following Breast Cancer Treatment: Discussing the Use of Soft Tissue Techniques. Physiotherapy. 2009; 95(4):314-320.

26. Leduc O, Sichere M, Moreau A, et al; Axillary web syndrome: nature and localisation. Lymphology. 2009;42(4): 176-81.

27. Whitley E, Bali J. Statistics review 4: sample size calculations. Crit Care (Bethesda). 2002;6:335-341.

28. Brazil. IBGE. Documentation and Information Dissemination Centre. Tabular presentation standards. IBGE. 3rd edition. Rio de Janeiro-RJ. 1993:62.

29. Steegers MA, Wolters B, Evers AW, et al. Effect of axillary lymph node dissection on prevalence and intensity of chronic and phantom pain after breast cancer surgery. J Pain. 2008;9:813-822.

30. Tasmuth T, von Smitten K, Hietanen P, et al. Pain and other symptoms after different treatment modalities of breast cancer. Ann Oncol. 1995;6:453-59.

31. Vinokur AD, Threatt BA, Vinokur-Kaplan D, et al. The process of recovery from breast cancer for younger and old patients. Changes during the first year. Cancer 1990;65:1242-54.

32. Leidenius M, Leivonen M, Vironen J, et al; The consequences of long-time arm morbidity in node-negative breast cancer patients with sentinel node biopsy or axillary clearance. J Surg Oncol. 2005;92:23-31.

33. Petrek JA, Senie RT, Peters M, et al; Lymphedema in a cohort of breast carcinoma survivors 20 years after diagnosis. Cancer. 2001 ;6:1368-1377.

34. Sagen Â, Kâresen R, Risberg MA. Physical activity for the affected limb and arm lymphedema after breast cancer surgery. A prospective, randomised controlled trial with two years follow-up. Acta Oncol. 2009;48:1 102-110.

35. Rõnkä RH, Pamilo MS, von Smitten KA, et al; Breast lymphedema after breast conserving treatment. Acta Oncol. 2004;6:551-57.

36. Fukushima KFP, Silva HJ, Ferreira CWS. Vascular changes resulting from the surgical approach to the axilla: A review of the literature. Rev Bras de Mastologia 2011;21(2):91-98.

37. Rodrigues, M. A. M.; Camargo, J. L. V. Carcinogenesis. In: Montenegro, M. F. *Et Al.* **Pathology General Processes.** 5th Ed. Chap 15. São Paulo: Ed. Atheneu, 2010. P. 255.

38. Jemal, A. *Et Al.* Global Cancer Statistics. **Ca: A Cancer Journal For Clinicians,** V. 61, N. 2, P. 134, 2011.

39. Chen, Y., Brock, G., Dongfeng, W. Estimating Key Parameters In Periodic Breast Cancer Screening - Application To The Canadian National Breast Screening Study Data. **Cancer Epidemiology,** Amsterdam, V. 34, N. 4, P. 429-433, Aug. 2010.

40. Polyak, K., Breast Cancer: Origins And Evolution. **The Journal Of Clinicai Investigation,** 117 (11), 2007.

41. Willis, L. *Et Al.* Breast Cancer Dormancy Can Be Maintained By Small Numbers Of Micrometastases. **Cancer Research,** 70: 4310-4317, 2010.

42. Globocan. Cancer Fact Sheet. **Breast Cancer Incidence And Mortality Worldwide In 2008.** 2008. Available at: <Http://Globocan.Iarc.Fr/Factsheets/Cancers/Breast.Asp>. Accessed on: 29/04/2012.

43. Althuis, M. D. *Et Al.* Global Trends In Breast Cancer Incidence And Mortality 1973-1997. **International Journal Of Epidemiology,** Oxford, v. 34, p. 405-412, Apr. 2005.

44. Erickson, V. S. *Et Al.* Arm Oedema in Breast Cancer Patients. **Journal Of National**

Cancer Institute, Oxford, V. 93, .N. 2, P. 96-111, 2001.

45. Barekati, Z. *Et Al.* Methylation Signature Of Lymph Node Metastases In Breast Cancer Patients. **Cancer,** London, V. 12, N. 244, P. l-8,Jun. 2012.

46. Vervoot, M. M. *Et Al.* Trends In The Usage Of Adjuvant Systemic Therapy For Breast Cancer In The Netherlands And Its Effect On Mortality. **British Journal Cancer,** V. 19, N. 2, P. 242-247, Jul, 2004.

47. Ewertz M, Jensen AB: **Late effects of breast cancer treatment and potentials for rehabilitation.** *Acta Oncol* 2011. *Volume: 50,* 2:187-193.

48. Lemevall, A. Imaging Of Axillary Lymph Nodes. **Acta Oncológica,** V, 39, N. 3, P. 277-281,2000.

49. Reiland-Smith, J. Diagnosis And Surgical Treatment Of Breast Cancer. **South Dakota Medicine,** Special Issue, P. 31-37, 2010.

50. Blichert-Toft, M. Axillary Surgery In Breast Cancer Management. Background, Incidence And Extent Of Surgery And Accurate Axillary Staging, Surgical Procedures. **Acta Oncológica,** London, V. 39, N. 3, P. 269-275, 2000.

51. Ivens, D. *Et Al.* Assessment Of Morbidity From Complete Axillary Dissection. **British Journal Of Cancer,** V. 66, N. 1, P. 136-138, 1992.

52. Hiller, D.; Chu, Q.D. Cxcr4 And Axillary Lymph Nodes: Review Of A Potential Biomarker For Breast Cancer Metastasis. **International Journal Of Breast Cancer,** Cairo, Article Id 420981, 2011.

53. Soerjomataram, I. *Et Al.* An OverView Of Prognostic Factors For Long-Term Survivors Of Breast Cancer. Breast **Cancer Research And Treatment,** V. 107, N. 3, P.

309-330, Feb, 2008.

54. Shih, Y. C. T. *Et Al.* Incidence, Treatment Costs, And Complications Of Lymphedema After Breast Cancer: A 2-Year Follow-Up Study. **Journal Of Clinical Oncology**, V. 12, P. 2001-2014, 2009.

55. Gerber, L. H. *Et Al.* Factors Predicting Clinically Significant Fatigue In Women Following Treatment For Primary Breast Cancer. **Support Care Cancer, Published Online,** Berlin, V.19, N. 10, P. 1581-1591, Oct. 2010.

56. Mota, D. D. C. F.; Pimenta, C. A. M. Fatigue in Patients with Advanced Cancer: Concept, Evaluation and Intervention. **Revista Brasileira De Cancerologia,** V. 48, N. 4, P. 577-583,2002.

57. Dabakuyo, T. S. *Et Al.* A Multicentre Cohort Study To Compare Quality Of Life In Breast Cancer Patients According To Sentinel Lymph Node Biopsy Or Axillary Lymph Node Dissection. **Annals Of Oncology,** Oxford, V. 20, N. 8, P. 1352-1361, Jan. 2009.

58. Silberman, A. W. *et al.* Comparative Morbidity Of Axillary Lymph Node Dissection And The Sentinel Lymph Node Technique. Implications For Patients With Breast Cancer. **Annals Of Surgery,** V. 240, N. 1, P. 1-6, 2004.

59. Kootstra, J. J. *Et Al.* Longitudinal Comparison Of Arm Morbidity In Stage I-Ii Breast Cancer Patients Treated With Sentinel Lymph Node Biopsy. Sentinel Lymph Node Biopsy Followed By Completion Lymph Node Dissection, Or Axillary Lymph Node Dissection. **Annals Of Surgical Oncology,** V. 17, N. 9, P. 2384-2394, 2010.

60. Levitt, S.H. Approaching The Axilla In Breast Cancer. **Acta Oncologica,** (39), N.3:

261-264, 2000.

61. Kwaan, J.H., Rappaport, I. Postoperative Brachial Plexus Palsy. A Study On The Mechanism. **Archives Of Surgery, V.** 101, N. 5, P. 612-5, 1970

62. Ben-David, B., Stahl, C. Prognosis Of Intraoperative Brachial Plexus Injury. A Review Of 22 Cases. **British Journal Of Anaesthesia,** London, V. 79, N. 4, P. 440- 5, Oct. 1997.

63. Oktem, O.; Oktay, K. Fertility Preservation For Breast Cancer Patients. **Seminars in Reproductive Medicine,** v. 27, p. 486-92, 2009.

64. Rayson, D. *Et Al.* Anthracycline-Traztuzumab Regimens For Her 2/ Neu Overexpressing Breast Cancer: Current Experience And Future Strategies. **Annals Of Oncology,** V. 19, P. 1530-1539, 2008.

65. Schover, L. R. Premature Ovarian Failure And Its Consequences: Vasomotor Symptoms, Sexuality, And Fertility. **Journal Of Clinical Oncology,** V. 26, P. 753- 758, 2008.

66. Darby, S. C. *Et Al.* Radiation-Related Heart Disease: Current Knowledge And Future Prospects. **International Journal Of Radiation Oncology Biology Physics,** Tarrytown, V. 76, N. 3, P. 656-665, Mar. 2010.

67. Lee, J. J.; Swain, S. M. Peripheral Neurophathy Induced By Micro-Tubule-Stabilising Agents. **Journal Of Clinical Oncology,** V. 24, P. 1633-42, 2006.

68. Johansson, S. *et al.* Brachial Plexopathy After Postoperative Radiotherapy Of Breast Cancer Patients. A Long-Term Follow-Up. **Acta Oncologica,** V. 39, N. 3, P. 373- 382, 2000.

69. Herskind, C. *Et Al.* Fibroblast Differentiation In Subcutaneous Fibrosis After

Postmastectomy Radiotherapy. **Acta Oncológica,** London, V.39, N.3, P. 383-388, 2000.

70. Senofsky, G. M. *Et Al.* Total Axillary Lymphadenectomy In The Management Of Breast Cancer. **Archives Of Surgery,** V. 126, P. 1336-1342, 1991.

71. Rõnka, R. H. *Et Al.* One-Year Morbidity After Sentinel Node Biopsy And Breast Surgery. **The Breast,** V.14, Pg. 28-36, 2005.

72. Mortimer, P. S. The Pathophysiology Of Lymphoedema. **Cancer,** V. 83, 12 Suppl American, P. 2798-2802, 1998.

73. Rockson, S. G. Diagnosis And Management Of Lymphatic Vascular Disease. **Journal Of The American College Of Cardiology,** V. 52, P. 799-806, 2008.

74. Lane, K. N. *et al.* Upper Extremity Lymphatic Function At Rest And During Exercise In Breast Cancer Survivors With And Without Lymphedema Compared With Healthy Controls. **Journal Of Applied Physiology,** V. 103, P. 917-925, 2007.

75. Mellor, R. H. *et al.* Enhanced cutaneous lymphatic network in the forearms of women with postmastectomy oedema. **Journal of Vascular Research,** v. 37, p. 501- 512, 2000.

76. Rõnka, R. H. *Et Al.* Breast Lymphedema After Breast Conserving Treatment. **Acta Oncologica,** V. 43, N. 6, P. 551-557, 2004.

77. Celebioglu, F. *Et Al.* Lymph Drainage Studied By Lymphoscintigraphy In The Arms After Sentinel Node Biopsy Compared With Axillary Lymph Node Dissection Following Conservative Breast Cancer Surgery. **Acta Radiologica,** Stockholm, V. 48, N. 5, P. 488-95, Jun. 2007.

78. Tengrup, I. *Et Al.* Army Morbidity After Breast-Conserving Therapy For Breast Cancer. **Acta Oncologica,** V. 39, N. 3, P. 393-397, 2000.

79. Herd-Smith, A. *Et Al.* Prognostic Factors For Lymphedema After Primary Treatment Of Breast Carcinoma. **Cancer,** New York, V. 92, N. 7, P. 1783-1787, Oct. 2001.

80. Hopwood, P. *Et Al.* Start Trial Management Grp [Group Author]. Comparison Of Patient-Reported Breast, Arm, And Shoulder Symptoms And Body Image After Radiotherapy For Early Breast Cancer: 5-Year Follow-Up In The Randomised Standardisation Of Breast Radiotherapy (Start) Trials. **The Lancet Oncology,** London, V. 11, N. 3, P. 231-240, Mar. 2010.

81. Senofsky, G. M. *Et Al.* Total Axillary Lymphadenectomy In The Management Of Breast Cancer. **Archives Of Surgery,** V. 126, P. 1336-1342, 1991.

82. Mittendorf, E. A. Lymphatic Interrupted: Do We Really Understand The Risks And Consequences? **Annals Of Surgical Oncology,** (16): 1768-1770, 2009.

83. Karakousis, C.P. Surgical Procedures And Lymphedema Of The Upper And Lower Extremity. **Journal Of Surgical Oncology,** V.93, P. 87-91, 2006.

84. Kuroi, K. *Et Al.* Evidence-Based Risk Factors For Seroma Formation In Breast Surgery. **Japanese Journal Of Clinical Oncology,** V. 36, N. 4, P. 197-206, 2006.

85. lovino, F. *Et Al.* Preventing Seroma Formation After Axillary Dissection For Breast Cancer: A Randomised Clinical Trial. **The American Journal Of Surgery,** New York, V. 203, Pg. 708-714, Jun. 2012.

86. Dalberg, K. *et al.* A Randomised Study Of Axillary Drained And Pectoralis Pectoris Preservation After Mastectomy For Breast Cancer. **The Journal Of Cancer Surgery,** London, V. 30, N. 6, P. 602-609, Aug. 2004.

87. Lovely, J. K. *Et Al.* Balancing Venous Thromboembolism And Haematoma After

Breast Surgery. **Annals Of Surgical Oncology**, V. 19, P. 3230-3235, 2012.

88. Jung, B. *et al.* Neuropathic Pain After Breast Cancer Surgery: Proposed Classification And Research Update. **Pain,** V. 104, P. 1-13, 2003.

89. Abdi, S.; Sheon, R.P. Etiology, Clinical Manifestations, And Diagnosis Of Complex Regional Pain Syndrome In Adults. <

<Http://Www.Uptodate.Com/Contents/Etiology-Clinical-Manifestations-And-Diagnosis-Of-Complex-Regional-Pain-Syndrome-In-Adults?Source=Search_Result&Search=Reflex+Sympathetic+Dystrophy&Selectedtit l e=l%7E53> > Accessed on 22/08/12.

90. Brooks, P.; Malic, C.; Austen, O. Intercostobrachial Nerve Injury From Axillary Dissection Resulting In Necrotizing Faciitis After A Burn Injury. **The Breast Journal,** Malden, V. 14, N. 2, 385-387, Jul./Aug. 2008.

91. Wallace, M. S. *Et Al.* Pain After Breast Surgery: A Survey Of 282 Women. **Pain,** V. 66, P. 195-205, 1996.

92. Reedijk M. Boemer S, Ghazarian D, et al; A case of axillary web syndrome with subcutaneous nodules following axillary surgery. *Breast.* 2006:411-413.

93. Rezende, L. F.; Franco R. L.; Gurgel, M. S. C. Axillary Web Syndrome: Practical Implications. **The Breast Journal,** V. 11, N. 6, P. 531, 2005.

94. Hung, S. S. J. Deep Vein Thrombosis Of The Arm Associated With Malignancy. **Cancer,** New York, V. 64, P. 531-535, 1989.

95. Queiroz, P. C. *Et Al.* Prevalence of Micro- and Macro-vascular Complications and Their Risk Factors in Patients with Diabetes *Mellitus* and Metabolic Syndrome. **Revista Brasileira De Clínica Medica,** São Paulo, V. 9, N. 4, P. 254-8, 2011.

96. Yugar-Toledo, J. C.; Moreno Júnior, H. Implications of Active Smoking and Passive Smoking as a Mechanism for Stabilising Atherosclerotic Plaque. **Revista da Sociedade de Cardiologia,** São Paulo, v. 12, n. 4, p. 595-605, 2002.

97. Aydogan, F. *Et Al.* C. Axillary Web Syndrome After Sentinel Node Biopsy. **Breast Care (Basel),** Switzerland, V. 3, N. 4, P. 277-278, 2008. Published Online, Aug. 2009.

CHAPTER 6

TABLES

Table 1 - Association between symptoms related to surgery and diagnosis of SARS in 97 women - Pernambuco Cancer Hospital - December 2011-July 2012

Report of post-surgical symptoms	SARS (cords) present (n=28)		absent (n=69)		p-value
	n	%	n	%	
Surgical scar pain					**0,003**
No	12	42,86	52	75,36	
Yes	16	57,14	17	24,64	
Pain in the armpit					0,302
No	16	57,14	45	65,22	
Yes	12	42,86	24	34,78	
Pain in the ipsilateral upper limb					**0,049**
No	17	60,71	55	79,71	
Yes	11	39,29	14	20,29	
Limited shoulder movement					0,119
No	6	21,43	25	36,23	
Yes	22	78,57	44	63,77	
Paresthesia reported in the ipsilateral upper limb					0,371
No	17	60,71	46	66,67	
Yes	11	39,29	23	33,33	
Paresis in the ipsilateral upper limb					0,445
No	9	32,14	25	36,23	
Yes	19	67,86	44	63,77	
Decreased strength in the ipsilateral upper limb*					0,348
No	15	55,56	33	48,53	
Yes	12	44,44	35	51,47	
Perception of cords No	12	42,86	51	73,91	**0,004**
Yes	16	57,13	18	26,09	
Pain on palpation of the cords^					0,417
No	3	18,75	5	27,78	
Yes	13	81,25	13	72,23	
Lightweight	5	38,46	8	61,54	
Moderate	5	38,46	3	23,08	
intense	3	23,08	2	15,38	

Note: * 95 patients reported a decrease in strength in the ipsilateral upper limb - percentage calculated on the number of patients who reported the perception of cords í P-value calculated using Chi-squared or Fisher's exact tests, according to frequency adequacy

Table 2- Means and standard errors of the mean age of the 97 patients according to symptoms related to surgery and diagnosis of SARS - Pernambuco Cancer Hospital - December 2011-July 2012

Report of surgery-related symptoms	Patient's age according to SARS (cords)				p-value
	average gift	(n=28) absent epm	medium (n=69)	epm	
Surgical scar pain	54,4	2,7	53,3	3,8	**0,021**
No	45,4	2,8	59,0	1,9	
Pain in the armpit	50,2	3,2	56,4	3,0	**0,021**
No	50,8	2,9	58,2	2,1	
Pain in the ipsilateral upper limb	53,6	3,1	52,2	3,0	**0,021**
No	48,6	2,8	59,0	2,0	
Limited shoulder movement	52,0	2,4	53,7	2,0	**0,021**
No	45,0	3,4	64,4	2,7	
Paresthesia reported in the ipsilateral upper limb	52,7	2,6	54,5	3,1	**0,021**
No	49,1	3,0	59,1	2,0	
Paresis reported in the ipsilateral upper limb	51,6	2,2	56,1	2,0	**0,021**
No	48,3	4,8	60,2	3,1	
Decreased strength in the ipsilateral upper limb*	49,8	3,8	54,4	2,5	**0,017**
No	50,6	2,5	61,2	2,3	
Perception of painful cords	53,0	2,9	56,8	4,2	0,377
No	38,7	4,3	47,6	4,5	

Caption: epm - standard error of the mean p-value calculated using Student's t-test for differences between means

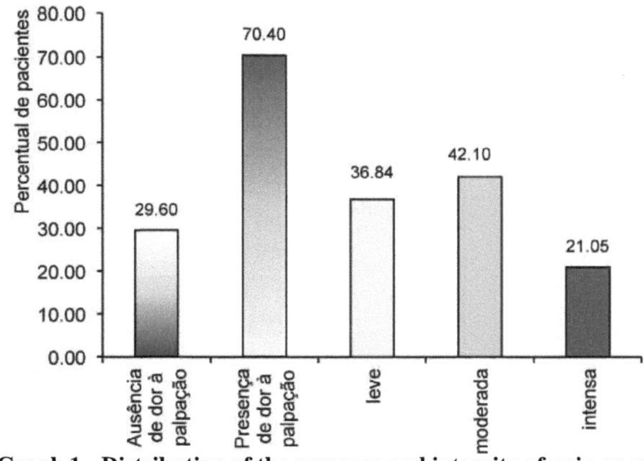

Graph 1 - Distribution of the presence and intensity of pain on palpation of the characteristic SARS cords in 16 women who reported perceiving the cords - Pernambuco Cancer Hospital - December 2011-July 2012

Table 3 - Distribution of the frequency of reduced active and passive shoulder movement according to 27 patients who reported pain on palpation of the characteristic SARS cords (cords) - Pernambuco Cancer Hospital - December 2011-July 2012

Reductions in movement assessed by goniometry	Pain on palpation of the cords				P-value
	present (n=19*)		absent (n=8)		
	n	%	n	%	
reduced active shoulder flexion	18	94,74	7	87,50	0,513
absent	1	5,26	1	12,50	
reduced active shoulder extension	12	63,16	5	62,5	0,651
absent	7	36,84	3	37,5	
reduction of active shoulder abduction	19	100,00	7	87,50	0,296
absent	-	-	1	12,5	
reduction of active shoulder adduction	12	63,16	5	62,5	0,651
absent	7	36,84	3	37,5	
reduction of active shoulder internal rotation	14	73,68	3	37,5	0,091
absent	5	26,32	5	62,5	
reduction of active external rotation of the shoulder	9	47,37	4	50,00	0,615
absent	10	52,63	4	50,00	
reduction of passive shoulder flexion	18	94,74	7	87,50	0,513
absent	1	5,26	1	12,5	
reduction of passive shoulder extension	11	57,90	4	50,00	0,516
absent	8	42,10	4	50,00	
reduction of passive shoulder abduction	19	100,00	7	87,50	0,296
absent	-	-	1	12,50	
reduction of passive shoulder adduction	10	52,64	4	50,00	0,615
absent	9	47,36	4	50,00	
reduction of passive internal rotation of the shoulder	15	78,94	5	62,50	0,332
absent	4	21,01	3	37,50	
reduction of passive external rotation of the shoulder	11	57,90	2	25,00	0,127
absent	8	42,10	6	75,00	

Note: p-values calculated using the Chi-squared or Fisher's exact test, according to frequency distribution * Data on pain was lost in one patient with SARS

Table 4 - Distribution of the frequency of reduced active and passive shoulder movement after breast cancer surgery according to SARS groups (cords) - Pernambuco Cancer Hospital - December 2011-July 2012

Reductions in movement assessed by goniometry	SARS present (n=28)		absent (n=69)		P-value
	n	%	n	%	
reduced active shoulder flexion	26	92,86	60	86,96	0,329
absent	2	7,14	9	13,04	
reduced active shoulder extension	18	64,28	36	52,17	0,195
absent	10	35,72	33	47,83	
reduction of active shoulder abduction	27	96,42	58	84,06	0,084
absent	1	3,58	11	15,94	
reduction of active shoulder adduction	17	60,71	36	52,17	0,295
absent	11	39,29	33	47,83	
reduction of active shoulder internal rotation	18	64,29	47	68,12	0,446
absent	10	35,71	22	31,88	
reduction of active external shoulder rotation	14	50,00	34	49,28	0,563
absent	14	50,00	35	50,72	
reduction of passive shoulder flexion	26	92,86	55	79,71	0,096
absent	2	7,14	14	20,29	
reduction of passive shoulder extension	16	57,14	32	46,38	0,231
absent	12	42,86	37	53,62	
reduction of passive shoulder abduction	27	96,43	55	79,71	**0,032**
absent	1	3,57	14	20,29	
reduction of passive shoulder adduction	14	50,00	30	43,48	0,359
absent	14	50,00	39	56,52	
reduction of passive internal rotation of the shoulder	20	71,43	46	66,66	0,420
absent	8	28,57	23	33,33	
reduction of passive external rotation of the shoulder	13	46,43	28	40,58	0,380
absent	15	53,57	41	59,42	

Note: p-values calculated using the Chi-squared or Fisher's exact test, according to frequency distribution

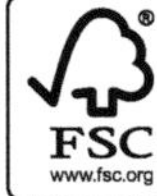

MIX
Papier aus verantwortungsvollen Quellen
Paper from responsible sources
FSC® C105338

FSC
www.fsc.org

Printed by Books on Demand GmbH, Norderstedt / Germany